Heart Disease: How to Reverse Heart Disease and Avoid a Heart Attack,

the Essential Guide to Diagnosis, Treatment and Prevention

Lazarus P. Hermanson

ACKNOWLEDGEMENT

I would like to thank my family and friends for their support and encouragement during the writing of this book. I am also grateful to my colleagues, who provided invaluable insights and feedback throughout the process. Finally, I extend my deepest appreciation to the medical professionals who have dedicated their lives to understanding and treating cardiovascular illness. Your knowledge and dedication to this field have been a great inspiration to me.

TABLE OF CONTENT

I. Introduction to Cardiovascular Disease

Heart disease is a wide word that refers to a variety of heart-related illnesses. It is the largest cause of death in America, accounting for one out of every four fatalities. Coronary artery disease, arrhythmias, heart defects, and heart failure are among disorders that might be classified as heart disease.

The most frequent kind of cardiac illness is coronary artery disease (CAD). Atherosclerosis happens when the arteries that feed blood to the heart become restricted or obstructed as a result of plaque development. This may result in chest discomfort, shortness of breath, and, in extreme cases, a heart attack. Arrhythmias are irregular heartbeats that may cause the heart to beat excessively quickly, too slowly, or irregularly. A range of variables, including genetics, drugs, and underlying cardiac diseases, may contribute to this.

Heart defects are structural cardiac disorders that may occur at birth or develop later in life. They may include heart holes, valve issues, and aberrant heart muscle.

Heart failure occurs when the heart is unable to pump enough blood to fulfill the demands of the body. This might result in weariness, shortness of breath, and leg and foot edema.

Heart disease is a dangerous ailment that may be fatal. It is important to identify the signs and symptoms of heart disease and get medical assistance if any of them occur. High blood pressure, high cholesterol, diabetes, smoking, obesity, and a sedentary lifestyle are all risk factors for heart disease.

Changes in lifestyle, such as eating a nutritious diet, exercising frequently, and stopping smoking, may help lower your chance of getting heart disease. Regular exams and screenings are also recommended to discover any possible concerns early.

Heart disease is a severe ailment with substantial consequences for your health and quality of life. Taking precautions and identifying the signs and symptoms of heart disease may help you remain healthy and lower your chance of acquiring this illness.

A. Heart Disease Definition

Heart disease is a wide phrase that refers to a variety of medical diseases that affect the heart or its blood arteries. These illnesses may be caused by several factors and result in a variety of symptoms. Heart illness may cause irregular heartbeats, blockages in the coronary arteries, and the heart's inability to adequately pump blood. Other disorders that may be involved include coronary artery disease, congestive heart failure, and stroke.

Heart disease is a leading cause of death in the United States and other parts of the globe. Heart disease is the top cause of mortality for both men and women in the United States. It is responsible for more than one-third of all deaths each year. Several factors contribute to heart disease, including smoking, obesity, high blood pressure, high cholesterol, and diabetes. Genetics and family history are important factors. Physical inactivity and poor diet are two more lifestyle variables that might contribute to the development of heart disease.

Depending on the situation, the signs and

symptoms of heart disease might vary. Chest discomfort, shortness of breath, exhaustion, and heart palpitations are some of the most prevalent symptoms. Also, those with heart problems may develop dizziness, nausea, and leg edema.

A medical history, physical exam, and several tests are used to diagnose cardiac disease. An electrocardiogram (ECG), echocardiography, and stress test are among the diagnostics available. Blood testing may also identify the presence of certain proteins that signal the existence of the cardiac disease.

Therapy for heart disease is condition-specific. It usually involves adjustments to one's lifestyle, such as stopping smoking, eating a nutritious diet, and exercising frequently. Medicines may also be provided to lower the risk of having a heart attack or a stroke. Surgery may be required in certain circumstances to unblock clogged coronary arteries. Heart disease is a dangerous disorder that may significantly reduce a person's quality of life. Making lifestyle modifications and visiting a doctor regularly may help minimize the risk of heart disease. People with heart disease may live long and active lives with the proper care and treatment.

B. Heart Disease Types

Heart disease is a wide phrase that refers to any ailment that affects the heart and its function. Heart illness may vary from simple issues like mitral valve prolapse to significant issues like coronary artery disease, which can lead to a heart attack and death. Heart disease is the biggest cause of mortality in the United States, with an estimated 600,000 People dying from it each year.
DISEASE OF THE CORONARY ARTERY (CAD)

The most frequent kind of cardiac illness is coronary artery disease. Coronary artery disease (CAD) is a prevalent and potentially fatal kind of heart disease. It is a disease in which the arteries supplying blood to the heart become obstructed or constricted. This may reduce blood supply to the heart, resulting in a range of symptoms and consequences such as chest discomfort (angina), heart attack, and heart failure. The most frequent kind of heart disease and the major cause of mortality in the United States and other industrialized nations is coronary artery disease (CAD).

Atherosclerosis, commonly known as artery stiffening, is the most prevalent cause of CAD. Atherosclerosis is the accumulation of fatty deposits (plaque) on the inner walls of the arteries. This may constrict or obstruct the arteries, lowering the quantity of blood that can flow through them. This may result in insufficient oxygen and nutrients reaching the heart, as well as a buildup of waste products.

High blood pressure, high cholesterol, smoking, diabetes, obesity, a family history of heart disease, age, and a sedentary lifestyle are all risk factors for CAD. Moreover, a diet heavy in saturated and trans fat, as well as a lack of Physical exercise may aid in the progression of CAD. Quitting smoking, exercising frequently, and eating a balanced diet are all part of CAD treatment. To lower the risk of a heart attack, medications such as aspirin, statins, and beta-blockers may be administered. Surgical techniques such as angioplasty or bypass surgery may be required in certain circumstances to restore blood flow to the heart.

CAD is a severe disorder that, if not treated appropriately, may be fatal. It is important to be aware of the risk factors and symptoms of CAD

and to get medical
attention if you encounter
any of them. If you have
any of the risk factors for
CAD, speak to your
doctor about how you
might lower your risk.

FAILURE OF THE HEART

Heart failure is another
prevalent kind of cardiac
illness in which the heart
is unable to pump enough
blood to satisfy the body's
demands. It is a
dangerous and possibly
fatal disease that affects
millions of individuals
globally. A range of
reasons, including
coronary artery disease,
high blood pressure,
diabetes, and other
illnesses, may lead to
heart failure.

Shortness of breath is the most frequent sign of heart failure, which may be followed by weariness, swelling in the legs and ankles, and a fast or irregular pulse.

Additional symptoms may include chest discomfort, dizziness, and an abdominal sense of fullness.

Heart failure therapy is determined by the underlying cause and the severity of the ailment. Lifestyle adjustments such as stopping smoking, eating a balanced diet, and exercising frequently may help improve symptoms in certain situations. Diuretics, ACE inhibitors, and beta-blockers are examples of medications that may be used to lower the burden on the heart and improve symptoms. In more severe situations, surgery to repair or replace damaged heart tissue may be required.

Heart failure may be a challenging illness to manage, but with the correct medication and lifestyle adjustments, symptoms and quality of life can be improved. Working with your doctor to design a treatment plan that is correct for you is essential. Frequent follow-up visits and condition monitoring are also necessary to verify that your therapy is successful.

Living with heart failure may be difficult, but there

are several tools available
to assist. Support groups,
instructional materials,
and other resources may
assist you in learning
more about the disorder
and how to manage it. It
is essential to bring up
any worries or queries
you have with your
physician. It is possible to
live a full and active life
with heart failure with the
correct care and
treatment.

DISEASE OF THE VALVULAR HEART

Valvular heart disease
occurs when one or more
of the heart valves fails to
function correctly. These
valves control the flow of
blood through the heart,
and when one or more of
them fails, it may lead to
major consequences.

Valvular heart disease
may be caused by a
variety of reasons,
including congenital
defects, aging, and
infections.
Aortic stenosis, or
narrowing of the aortic
valve, is the most
frequent kind of valvular
heart disease. This is
caused by calcium
deposits, which may
accumulate over time and
limit the size of the
aperture. Congenital
defects, rheumatic heart
disease, and endocarditis,
an infection of the inner
lining of the heart, are
some of the other reasons
for aortic stenosis. Chest
discomfort, shortness of
breath, and exhaustion
may all be symptoms of
aortic stenosis.

Another kind of valvular heart disease is mitral valve prolapse. This happens when the mitral valve, which controls blood flow between the left atrium and the left ventricle, swells and bulges into the left atrium. This may result in mitral regurgitation, a disease in which blood rushes back into the atrium rather than forward into the ventricle. Palpitations, chest discomfort, and shortness of breath are all symptoms of mitral valve prolapse.

Another kind of valvular heart disease is tricuspid valve regurgitation. This happens when the tricuspid valve, which connects the right atrium to the right ventricle, gets overly broad, allowing blood to flow back into the right atrium. Tricuspid valve regurgitation symptoms include weariness, palpitations, and shortness of breath.

Lastly, aortic regurgitation occurs when the aortic valve fails to seal correctly, allowing some blood to flow back into the left ventricle. This may result in congestive heart failure, a dangerous and sometimes fatal disease. Aortic regurgitation symptoms include chest discomfort, shortness of breath, and weariness.

The kind and severity of valvular heart disease will determine the course of treatment. Medication may be used to enhance the function of the valve in certain circumstances, while surgery may be required to repair or replace the defective valve in others. Nevertheless, lifestyle modifications including stopping smoking, exercising frequently, and eating a balanced diet may assist to lower the chance of getting valvular heart disease.

Valvular heart disease is a dangerous ailment that, if left untreated, may lead to catastrophic problems. As a result, if you have any signs of valvular heart disease, you should consult your doctor. The illness is typically effectively controlled with the right diagnosis and therapy.

CONGENITAL HEART DEFICIENCIES (CHDS)

Congenital heart defects (CHDs) are a collection of congenital anomalies that damage the structure of the heart. It is the most prevalent form of birth defect in the United States, affecting around one in every hundred births. CHDs are caused by faulty heart or major blood vessel development before birth. While the specific origin of CHDs is unclear, various risk factors, such as family history, viral infections, certain medicines, and environmental exposures, have been discovered.

Atrial septal defects (ASDs), ventricular septal defects (VSDs), and patent ductus arteriosus are the most prevalent kinds of CHDs (PDA). ASDs are holes in the heart's two upper chambers. VSDs are holes in the heart's two bottom chambers. PDA is a link between the pulmonary artery and the aorta that is abnormal. Pulmonary stenosis, tetralogy of Fallot, transposition of the major arteries, and truncus arteriosus are all examples of CHDs. Prenatal imaging can detect the majority of CHDs before birth. Echocardiography is frequently used to confirm the diagnosis after delivery. Treatment options may include drugs, minimally invasive treatments, or open-heart surgery, depending on the kind and severity of the abnormality. Complications from CHDs include heart failure, arrhythmias, stroke, and pulmonary hypertension. These consequences might be fatal in extreme circumstances. Early detection and treatment may lessen the likelihood of long-term problems. Living with CHDs may be difficult. It may have an impact on both physical and mental well-being, as well as academic achievement. Special adjustments may be required for children with CHDs to participate in school and other activities.

CHDs may have long-term consequences for people who suffer from them, although breakthroughs in diagnosis, therapy, and supportive care have improved results for many patients. Many individuals with CHDs may live full and productive lives with the right treatment and support.

ARRHYTHMIAS

Arrhythmias are abnormal heart rhythms that may occur in both healthy and sick persons. These irregular rhythms may cause the heart to beat excessively slowly, too fast, or in an uneven pattern. Arrhythmias are classified as supraventricular or ventricular. Supraventricular arrhythmias affect the heart's upper chambers, while ventricular arrhythmias affect the bottom chambers. Atrial fibrillation is the most prevalent kind of arrhythmia (AFib). This occurs when the heart rate is excessively high and the atria of the heart tremble rather than contract correctly. AFib may be caused by a variety of medical factors, including excessive blood pressure, thyroid illness, and heart valve issues. Palpitations, shortness of breath, dizziness, and exhaustion are all symptoms of AFib. Bradycardia, or a sluggish heart rate, is another frequent arrhythmia. An underlying medical condition, drugs, or even a healthy lifestyle might all contribute to this. Fatigue, fainting, dizziness, and shortness of breath are all symptoms of bradycardia. Ventricular arrhythmias are more dangerous and may result in cardiac arrest. Arrhythmias of this class include ventricular tachycardia (VT) and ventricular fibrillation (VF). When the heart beats excessively fast, it causes VT, which may induce chest discomfort, lightheadedness, and fainting. VF occurs when the heart quivers instead of beating properly and may result in chest discomfort, dizziness, and fainting.

Arrhythmia treatment is determined by the kind and severity of the arrhythmia as well as the underlying cause. Treatment alternatives include lifestyle changes such as stress reduction, avoidance of certain drugs, and eating a balanced diet. Medicines may also be used to assist manage the pace or rhythm of the heart. Surgery or device implantation may be required in certain circumstances to repair the arrhythmia.

Arrhythmias may be serious and even deadly. If you have any signs of arrhythmia, you should see your doctor right away since early detection and treatment may help avoid more severe problems.

PERICARDITIS

Pericarditis is an infection of the pericardium, which is the thin sac-like membrane that surrounds the heart and other critical organs. It is distinguished by inflammation, swelling, and irritation, which may result in chest discomfort, trouble breathing, and other unpleasant symptoms. A variety of events may contribute to it, including viral or bacterial infections, autoimmune illnesses, heart attacks, radiation treatment, renal failure, or trauma.

The most frequent pericarditis symptom is chest discomfort, which is often severe and stabbing and may be felt on either side of the chest cavity. Tenderness in the left shoulder, neck, and arms is also possible. Fever, shortness of breath, exhaustion, and a sense of heaviness in the chest are other frequent symptoms. The disorder may also cause an irregular pulse and palpitations in certain people.

Depending on the underlying cause, pericarditis is often treated with pharmaceuticals such as anti-inflammatory agents and antibiotics. Surgery may be required in rare circumstances to remove excess fluid or scar tissue from the pericardium. In extreme situations, a pericardiectomy to remove the whole pericardium may be needed.

Pericarditis, if left untreated, may result in consequences such as cardiac tamponade, a potentially fatal disease in which the heart is unable to pump properly owing to excessive fluid collection in the pericardium. It may also induce constrictive pericarditis, which occurs when the pericardium stiffens and inhibits the heart from filling with blood.

If you have any of the symptoms of pericarditis, you should seek medical attention right once to prevent complications. Early detection and treatment may assist to lower the risk of significant consequences and facilitate recovery. A healthy lifestyle, including regular exercise and a diet low in saturated fats and salt, is also essential. By taking these precautions, you may help to lower your chance of having pericarditis.

CARDIOMYOPATHY

Cardiomyopathy is a disorder in which the heart muscle enlarges, thickens, and/or becomes inflexible. It is a gradual, degenerative illness that impairs the capacity of the heart to pump blood, resulting in heart failure and associated consequences. Cardiomyopathy is a prominent cause of mortality in the United States, affecting between 1 in 500 and 1 in 2000 persons. Cardiomyopathy's specific source is unclear, however, it may be caused by several causes such as genetic defects, viral infections, metabolic problems, and environmental pollutants. High blood pressure, diabetes, and obesity are other risk factors. Cardiomyopathy may be classified into numerous categories. The most frequent kind is dilated cardiomyopathy, in which the heart's walls become stretched and thin, making it difficult for the heart to pump blood properly. The second most frequent kind is hypertrophic cardiomyopathy, in which the heart muscle thickens, making it harder for the heart to relax and fill with blood. Restrictive cardiomyopathy occurs when the heart's walls stiffen, restricting the heart's capacity to fill with blood. Cardiomyopathy symptoms vary based on the kind and severity of the ailment. Shortness of breath, chest discomfort, tiredness, and palpitations

are common symptoms.
Arrhythmia, heart failure,
and sudden cardiac death
are all possible
complications.
A physical examination,
medical history, lab
testing, and imaging tests
such as an
echocardiography or MRI
are used to diagnose
cardiomyopathy. Therapy
for cardiomyopathy
might involve lifestyle
modifications, drugs,
surgery, and/or device
treatment, depending on
the kind.
Quitting smoking,
reducing alcohol intake,
eating a nutritious diet,
and exercising frequently
are all examples of
lifestyle modifications.
Diuretics are used to
decrease fluid in the

body, ACE inhibitors to lower blood pressure, and beta-blockers to lower heart rate and blood pressure. If drugs and lifestyle modifications are ineffective, surgery may be required. Pacemakers, defibrillators, and implanted cardioverter defibrillators are examples of device treatment.

Cardiomyopathy is a dangerous ailment that, if not treated appropriately, may be fatal. It is critical for those suffering from cardiomyopathy to follow their doctor's advice and take all medicines as directed. It is also critical to maintaining a healthy lifestyle, which includes eating a balanced diet, exercising frequently, and refraining from smoking and excessive alcohol usage. Cardiomyopathy patients may live normal life with correct therapy and lifestyle changes. Finally, there are several forms of cardiac disease. Some are trivial, while others are potentially fatal. It is important to recognize the signs and risk factors for heart disease and to get treatment if required. You may lower your chances of acquiring a major cardiac issue by doing so.

II. Heart Disease Causes

Heart disease is a broad phrase that encompasses a wide range of heart-related disorders, including coronary artery disease, congestive heart failure, irregular heart rhythms, and congenital heart abnormalities. Heart disease is the leading cause of mortality and a significant source of disability in the United States. Knowing the causes of heart disease is critical for preventing and treating it.

Genetics

Heart disease development may be influenced by genetics and family history. Certain hereditary illnesses, such as familial hypercholesterolemia, may result in elevated blood cholesterol levels. Some genetic diseases, such as Marfan's syndrome, may result in structural changes in the heart and blood arteries. Several disorders may raise one's chances of acquiring heart disease.

Exercise and Diet

The things we consume may have a direct impact on our cardiovascular health. Consuming a diet heavy in saturated fat and cholesterol may raise blood levels of these chemicals, increasing the risk of developing heart disease. A diet rich in fruits and vegetables, healthy grains, and lean meats may help decrease cholesterol and minimize the risk of heart disease. Physical activity and exercise are also beneficial to cardiovascular health. Exercise regularly may help decrease blood pressure, lower cholesterol levels, and enhance overall cardiovascular health. Individuals who engage in physical activity have a decreased chance of acquiring heart disease.

Smoking

Tobacco use is a significant risk factor for heart disease. Smoking may cause artery lining damage, which can lead to plaque formation. This may cause artery narrowing and raise the risk of a heart attack or stroke. Smoking also raises the likelihood of having high blood pressure, which is a risk factor for heart disease.

Blood Pressure Is Excessive

High blood pressure is a significant risk factor for heart disease. High blood pressure may cause the artery walls to thicken and stiffen, resulting in plaque formation. This may cause artery narrowing and raise the risk of a heart attack or stroke.

Diabetes

Diabetes is a disease in which the body's ability to manage the quantity of sugar in the blood is impaired. Diabetes puts people at a higher risk of developing heart disease because high blood sugar levels may damage artery walls and raise the chance of a heart attack or stroke.

Obesity

Obesity is a significant risk factor for

cardiovascular disease. Obesity and overweight raise the risk of getting high blood pressure, high cholesterol, and diabetes. Any of these disorders might raise your chances of getting heart disease.

Stress

Stress may be harmful to one's heart health. Stress causes the body to create chemicals like adrenaline and cortisol, which raise blood pressure and heart rate. This may raise the chance of getting heart disease.

Age

Our chance of acquiring heart disease rises as we age. This is because risk factors for heart disease, such as high blood pressure, high cholesterol, and diabetes, grow more prevalent as people age. Moreover, the arteries might stiffen and constrict, increasing the risk of a heart attack or stroke.

Gender

Males are more prone than women to getting heart disease. This is because males have greater cholesterol levels and are more prone to lead sedentary lifestyles. Men are also more likely to smoke and have risk conditions such as high blood pressure and diabetes.

Race

Some racial and ethnic groupings are more likely to acquire heart disease. High blood pressure and diabetes are more common among Black

Americans, Native Americans, and Hispanic Americans, which may raise the risk of developing heart disease. Black Americans are also more likely to have a family history of heart disease.

Knowing the causes of heart disease is critical for preventing and treating it. Genetics and family history are two risk factors for heart disease that cannot be avoided. Other risk factors, such as diet and exercise, smoking, and stress, may, however, be treated and controlled to lower the chance of getting heart disease.

III. Heart Disease Signs

Heart disease is a wide word that refers to a variety of heart-related illnesses. It is the top cause of death in the United States and worldwide. Heart disease symptoms vary based on the kind of ailment, but the most frequent signs and symptoms include chest discomfort, shortness of breath, exhaustion, irregular heartbeat, and swelling in the legs and feet.

Chest Ache

Chest discomfort is a typical sign of heart disease that may be caused by several different illnesses.

Coronary artery disease, which is the narrowing of the arteries that feed blood to the heart, is the most prevalent cause of chest discomfort. This constriction may reduce the quantity of oxygen and nutrients reaching the heart muscle, resulting in chest discomfort. Heart attacks, angina, pericarditis, and pulmonary embolism are among illnesses that may cause chest discomfort. A total blockage of a coronary artery causes a heart attack. This obstruction may harm the heart muscle, and the discomfort is often characterized as a crushing or squeezing sensation in the chest. Angina is a kind of chest discomfort produced by a narrowing of the coronary arteries, which may reduce the amount of oxygen and nutrients reaching the heart muscle. Pericarditis is an infection of the sac that surrounds the heart that may produce stabbing discomfort in the chest. A pulmonary embolism is a blood clot that moves to the lungs, causing chest discomfort, shortness of breath, and an irregular pulse.

It is important to see a doctor and undergo a physical exam to determine the source of chest discomfort. Further tests, such as an electrocardiogram, echocardiography, heart stress test, or angiography, may be ordered by the doctor. An ECG detects heart attacks by measuring the electrical activity of the heart. An echocardiogram creates an image of the heart using sound waves and may be used to diagnose heart valve issues or irregular heart rhythms. A cardiac stress test is used to determine how effectively the heart reacts to physical exercise and may aid in the diagnosis of coronary artery disease. Angiography is a kind of imaging procedure that looks for blockages in the coronary arteries using X-rays and contrast dye. The treatment for chest discomfort caused by heart disease is determined by the underlying cause. If coronary artery disease is the root reason, lifestyle adjustments such as stopping smoking, exercising frequently, and eating a balanced diet are critical. Beta-blockers, ACE inhibitors, and statins may also help minimize the risk of a heart attack or stroke. If you have a heart attack, therapies like angioplasty and stenting may help free up clogged arteries and restore blood flow to your heart.

Chest pain may be a terrifying experience, but it is essential to realize that the majority of episodes of chest discomfort are not caused by heart disease. It is essential to see a doctor if you are experiencing chest discomfort and to seek medical assistance if the pain does not subside after a few minutes. The majority of instances of chest discomfort caused by heart disease may be adequately treated with the correct diagnosis and therapy.

Breathing Difficulty

Shortness of breath is a sign of heart disease, a medical condition. It is mainly caused by the heart's inability to pump oxygen-rich blood to the body's organs and tissues. Heart disease is a wide word that refers to a variety of medical diseases affecting the heart. Several disorders may induce decreased blood flow, resulting in symptoms such as shortness of breath.

A multitude of variables, including lifestyle choices, genetics, and age, may contribute to heart disease. Smoking, a poor diet, and a lack of exercise may all raise your chance of getting heart disease. Risk factors for heart disease include high blood pressure, high cholesterol, diabetes, and obesity. Genetics may also play a role since certain families are predisposed to develop heart disease. Age may also be a problem, as the body's ability to pump blood and oxygen across the body declines.

Heart disease, regardless of its etiology, may have

catastrophic implications. One of the most prevalent signs of heart disease is shortness of breath, which suggests a diminished capacity of the heart to pump oxygen-rich blood to the body's organs and tissues. It is often accompanied by chest discomfort, weariness, and dizziness. Additional signs of cardiac illness include irregular heartbeats, shortness of breath during physical exertion, and leg and foot edema.

The treatment for cardiac disease is determined by the underlying cause as well as the degree of the problem. Quitting smoking and adopting a healthy diet, for example, may help minimize the risk of heart disease. Blood pressure and cholesterol levels may be reduced using medications such as ACE inhibitors, beta-blockers, and diuretics. In more severe situations, surgery such as a coronary artery bypass graft (CABG) or valve replacement may be needed.

Shortness of breath might indicate a significant health issue such as heart disease. It is critical to get medical assistance if you suffer shortness of breath or any other signs of heart disease. Your doctor can assist you in determining the reason and administering the right therapy. With quick diagnosis and treatment, you can lower your chances of developing more severe heart disease problems.

Fatigue

Fatigue is a typical symptom of several illnesses, including heart disease. It may be physically and psychologically exhausting, making everyday tasks challenging. Several causes may contribute to fatigue, including a lack of sleep, physical exercise, or stress. It is also a typical indication of heart disease, a severe and sometimes fatal ailment.

Heart disease is a wide phrase that refers to any disorder that impairs the heart's capacity to operate normally. Conditions such as coronary artery disease, heart attack, and congestive heart failure are included. While symptoms vary by individual, weariness is a typical sign of heart disease.

Heart disease-related fatigue may be both physical and mental. A person suffering from heart disease may feel fatigued, weak, and depleted of vitality. They may find it difficult to do typical tasks and to remain up for more than a few hours at a time. A person suffering from heart disease may have difficulties focusing, memory issues, and mood changes.

Fatigue in heart disease is caused by several factors.

It may be caused by a variety of circumstances, including drug side effects, physical effort, or the illness itself. Heart disease medications may produce sleepiness, low energy levels, and weariness. Physical effort may also create exhaustion, particularly if the individual is not accustomed to exercising or engaging in physical activities. Lastly, the condition might produce weariness as a result of reduced blood flow to the heart muscle, which can result in lower oxygen levels in the body.

It is critical to determine the underlying cause of tiredness in heart disease before treating it. If it is drug-related, a doctor may help you decrease the dosage or switch to a different kind of medicine. If physical exercise causes weariness, it is critical to identify strategies to minimize activity levels and take more rest during the day. If the exhaustion is caused by the heart condition, lifestyle adjustments such as eating a balanced diet, exercising frequently, and minimizing stress may help.

Fatigue may be a debilitating sign of heart disease, but it is vital to remember that it is treatable. It is feasible to manage tiredness and live a more full life by recognizing the source of exhaustion and

implementing easy
lifestyle modifications.
Heartbeat Irregularity
Irregular heartbeat, often
known as arrhythmia, is a
cardiac rhythm problem
in which the heart beats
too slowly, too fast, or
irregularly. It affects
around 1 in every 100
persons and is more
frequent in women and as
people become older.
Heart palpitations, a
sense of a fast,
hammering, or fluttering
feeling in the chest, are
the most prevalent
indication of an irregular
heartbeat. Shortness of
breath, dizziness, chest
discomfort, exhaustion,
and fainting are some of
the other symptoms.
An irregular heartbeat is
often caused by an

underlying medical problem such as excessive blood pressure, coronary artery disease, or diabetes. An irregular heartbeat may be caused by a structural issue with the heart, such as a weaker heart muscle or faulty heart valves, in certain circumstances. Arrhythmias may also be caused by some medicines, including several over-the-counter medications.

Atrial fibrillation is the most frequent kind of abnormal heartbeat (AFib). This is a fast, irregular heartbeat that begins in the heart's upper chambers, known as the atria. AFib may cause blood to pool in the atria and clot, potentially leading to a stroke. Ventricular tachycardia is a less frequent kind of irregular heartbeat (VT). This is a quick, regular heartbeat that begins in the ventricles, the lowest chambers of the heart. VT may cause the heart to pump blood inefficiently, potentially resulting in a heart attack.

A doctor may first do a physical exam and order tests to discover the cause of an irregular heartbeat before treating it. Therapy may involve behavioral changes such as stress reduction and abstaining from alcohol and caffeine, as well as drugs such as beta-blockers and calcium channel blockers.

To treat an irregular heartbeat, a pacemaker or implanted cardioverter-defibrillator (ICD) may be required in certain circumstances. A pacemaker is a tiny device that transmits electrical impulses to the heart to keep it beating regularly. An ICD is a cardiac rhythm monitoring device that is placed in the chest. If the gadget identifies an aberrant beat, an electric shock is delivered to the heart to restore normal rhythm.

In addition to medical therapy, lifestyle changes may be required to assist manage an irregular heartbeat. Quitting smoking, eating a nutritious diet, exercising frequently, avoiding alcohol and caffeine, and minimizing stress are all examples.

An irregular heartbeat is a dangerous disorder that may lead to major complications such as stroke or heart attack. If you have any indications or symptoms of an abnormal heartbeat, you should see your doctor. Your doctor can advise you on the best therapy for your specific ailment.

Leg and foot swelling

Leg and foot swelling is a typical indication of cardiac disease. Edema, or swelling, is caused by an accumulation of fluid in the tissues. This fluid accumulation is produced by an abnormal accumulation of fluid in the body, which is mainly caused by impaired circulation.

Coronary artery disease is the most frequent kind of heart disease (CAD). A coronary artery disease (CAD) is a constriction of the blood channels that provide oxygen-rich blood to the heart muscle. When the blood supply to the heart is limited, the heart is unable to pump enough blood to the body, which causes the body to retain fluids. This fluid accumulation produces swelling in the legs and feet, which may be quite unpleasant.

Congestive heart failure (CHF) and valvular heart disease are two more types of heart disease that may cause edema in the legs and feet. CHF occurs when the heart is unable to pump enough blood to fulfill the body's demands. This causes fluid accumulation in the body, resulting in swelling in the legs and feet. Valvular heart disease is a disorder in which one or more of the heart's valves become damaged or weakened, causing fluid to accumulate in the body. Some lifestyle factors may raise the risk of heart disease and contribute to the development of edema. Poor diet, lack of exercise, smoking, and excessive alcohol use are examples of these. Diabetes, high blood pressure, and high cholesterol are all medical problems that might raise the chance of developing heart disease. It is essential to maintain a healthy lifestyle to prevent the risk of developing edema in the legs and feet as a result of heart disease. Consuming a well-balanced diet, exercising frequently, and abstaining from smoking and excessive alcohol intake may all help to lower the risk of getting heart disease. Moreover, controlling medical disorders such as diabetes, high blood pressure, and high cholesterol might help lower the chance of getting heart disease.

It is critical to get medical assistance if you are experiencing swelling in your legs and feet as a result of heart disease. To lower the chance of developing heart disease and the accompanying swelling in the legs and feet, your doctor may prescribe lifestyle modifications, drugs, or other therapies.

Surgery may be required in certain circumstances to address heart problems. Those with severe or advanced cardiac disease, or those who have not responded to lifestyle modifications and drugs, are usually advised to undergo surgery.

Finally, swelling in the legs and feet is a typical sign of cardiac disease. If you are having this symptom, you must keep a healthy lifestyle and get medical assistance. Adopting lifestyle changes, controlling medical problems, and taking medicines may all help lower the chance of getting heart disease and the swelling in the legs and feet that comes with it. Surgery may be required in certain circumstances to address heart problems.

If you see any of these symptoms, you should seek medical assistance immediately. Your doctor may undertake tests to establish the source of your symptoms and treat you accordingly.

IV. Diagnosis of Heart Disease

Diagnosis of heart disease is an essential element of preventive medicine and is necessary for efficient treatment. Diagnosis of heart disease may be challenging and requires a variety of diagnostic tests, imaging studies, and other information. The first step in diagnosing heart illness is to gather the patient's comprehensive medical history. This includes inquiries about lifestyle, a family history of cardiovascular disease, and any current symptoms or signs of heart disease. A physical examination may also be performed, which may provide further information about the patient's general health as well as any signs of heart illness.

The next step in the diagnosis of heart illness is diagnostic testing. These examinations include electrocardiograms (ECGs), echocardiograms, stress tests, and cardiac catheterizations. These tests might provide information about the patient's heart rate, rhythm, and function. They may also help discover arterial irregularities or blockages.

CT scans and magnetic resonance imaging (MRI)

scans may also be used to diagnose heart illness. These scans may offer physicians comprehensive pictures of the heart and surrounding tissue, enabling them to detect any abnormalities or blockages.

A heart disease diagnosis may sometimes be determined without the use of any testing or imaging techniques. A clinical diagnosis is formed by the doctor based on the patient's medical history, physical examination, and any additional signs and symptoms that the patient may be experiencing.

The doctor may prescribe the best therapy when a heart disease diagnosis has been obtained. Treatment for heart disease may involve dietary modifications, medicines, and, in rare circumstances, surgery. The degree and kind of cardiac disease influence the method of therapy. Early identification and treatment of heart illness may significantly reduce the risk of complications and perhaps improve the patient's quality of life. As a result, it is important to be aware of the signs and symptoms of heart disease and to get medical attention if you notice any of them.

A. Physical Exam

A physical examination for heart disease is an

important diagnostic and treatment method for cardiovascular illnesses. It includes a basic physical examination as well as a cardiovascular assessment. A physical examination may reveal anomalies that suggest underlying cardiac disease, such as abnormal heart sounds, murmurs, or pulses. This information may help to direct diagnostic testing and treatment even more precisely.

The patient's overall appearance, vital signs, skin, head and neck, chest, cardiovascular system, abdomen, limbs, and the neurologic system should all be evaluated during the general physical examination.

Blood pressure, pulse rate, and breathing rate are important indications of a patient's overall health and should be measured at every visit. On the skin, check for pallor, cyanosis, clubbing, edema, and other signs of heart failure. In the head and neck, examine for jugular venous distention, carotid bruits, and thyroid enlargement.

The chest symmetry, the presence of any masses or anomalies, and the presence of any cardiac rubs or murmurs should all be checked. Deep breathing and a Valsalva technique should be performed on the patient to detect murmurs.

Carotid artery bruits,

heart rate, rhythm, and any cardiovascular system murmurs should all be evaluated. In the belly, search for an abdominal aortic aneurysm. Edema, pulses, and pain or deformity in all four limbs should be assessed. The neurologic system should explore any signs of peripheral neuropathy.

In addition to the regular physical exam, a cardiovascular test should be performed. This includes examining the peripheral and carotid arterial pulses. The carotid pulse should be evaluated for a normal or irregular rate and rhythm, as well as any bruits. The peripheral pulse rate, rhythm, and volume should be assessed. It is critical to recognize the presence of an apical pulse. Any precordium lifts, heaves, thrills, or displacement should be explored. The heart should be auscultated for rate, rhythm, and cardiac sounds. Murmurs should be assessed based on their timing, place, strength, and length.

The physical examination for the cardiac disease may give important information for diagnosis and treatment. It should be done at every visit to look for any new or altering results. The physical exam, when performed properly, may reveal underlying cardiac disease and lead to further diagnostic tests and therapy.

B. Blood Test

Blood tests are often used to diagnose heart disease, identify risk factors for heart disease, evaluate therapy efficacy, and measure overall heart health. Tests may be performed to determine the levels of cholesterol, triglycerides, lipoproteins, liver enzymes, thyroid hormones, and clotting hormones, as well as electrolytes and other chemicals. Tests may also be performed to determine the oxygen content of the blood and to identify the presence of certain immune system markers.

C. Imaging Exams

Imaging tests are useful in detecting and monitoring heart disease because they enable physicians to observe the architecture of the heart and veins as well as the flow of blood through them. Echocardiogram, computed tomography (CT) scan, magnetic resonance imaging (MRI), nuclear imaging, and cardiac catheterization are the most frequent imaging techniques used to diagnose and monitor heart illness.
A form of ultrasonography is

echocardiography. It creates pictures of the heart using sound waves, including the chambers, valves, walls, and blood arteries that link to it. It may aid in the diagnosis of illnesses such as cardiomyopathy and valve issues.

A computed tomography (CT) scan is a kind of X-ray that looks at the heart and chest. A CT scan may reveal blockages in the coronary arteries as well as other cardiac problems.

Magnetic resonance imaging (MRI) creates comprehensive pictures of the heart and blood arteries by using a strong magnetic field and radio waves. It is used to identify cardiac muscle degeneration, heart valve anomalies, and coronary artery blockages. Nuclear imaging is a sort of imaging examination that employs a radioactive tracer to assess heart function. This test may discover parts of the heart that are not receiving enough blood flow as a result of blockages or constricted arteries.

A thin, flexible tube (catheter) is placed into an artery in the arm, groin, or neck and threaded through the blood arteries to the heart during cardiac catheterization. Dye is injected into the coronary arteries during the treatment to assist surgeons to view the arteries and discover any blockages.

Imaging studies are useful for detecting and monitoring heart disease because they allow clinicians to identify the degree of the illness and design the best therapy for the patient. They may also aid in the early detection of abnormalities, lowering the risk of complications.

V. Heart Disease Therapy

Heart illness is a wide term encompassing a variety of disorders that affect the heart or its blood arteries. It is one of the major causes of mortality and disability in the world today, and

people who suffer from it
may face substantial
long-term effects.

A. Changes in Lifestyle

Lifestyle modifications
are an important part of
controlling heart disease
and avoiding
complications. The goal
of this article is to
describe how adopting
lifestyle changes might
assist persons with heart
disease and lessen the
chance of subsequent
issues.
Implementing lifestyle
modifications may
improve the health of
people with heart disease.
A heart-healthy lifestyle
begins with eating a
healthy, balanced diet.

Consuming a variety of fruits and vegetables, complete grains, and lean meats may assist in lowering cholesterol and maintaining a healthy weight. Reducing saturated and trans fats, and salt, and limiting processed meals and sugary beverages may all help to lower your risk of heart disease.

Another significant lifestyle modification for patients with heart disease is regular physical exercise. Exercise may help lower blood pressure and cholesterol levels while also improving cardiac strength and fitness. To promote overall cardiovascular health, aim for at least 30 minutes of moderate physical exercise most days of the week.

Stopping smoking is another crucial lifestyle modification for persons suffering from heart disease. Smoking raises the chance of having a heart attack, a stroke, or developing other cardiovascular disorders. Stopping smoking may lower the chance of future difficulties while also improving overall heart health.

Stress management is also an important lifestyle modification for those with heart disease. Since stress increases the risk of heart attack and stroke, it is important to take actions to minimize stress levels. Getting adequate sleep, practicing relaxation methods, and participating in regular physical exercise are all strategies to alleviate stress.

Lastly, other health disorders that might raise the risk of heart diseases, such as diabetes and high blood pressure, must be managed. Collaboration with a healthcare professional to treat these problems and make any required lifestyle adjustments may help lower the chance of additional issues.

In conclusion, implementing lifestyle modifications may improve the health of those with heart disease. Consuming a healthy, balanced diet, exercising regularly, stopping smoking, managing stress, and controlling other health concerns may all help to lower the chance of additional difficulties and improve overall heart health.

B. Pharmaceuticals

Medication is an essential component of any heart disease treatment regimen. These may help lower the chances of having a heart attack, stroke, or another cardiovascular event, as well as control symptoms and enhance the overall quality of life. Based on the type and severity of your heart condition, your doctor may suggest one or more of the drugs listed below.

1. **Cholesterol-lowering drugs:** High cholesterol is a key risk factor for heart disease, and drugs like statins may help decrease cholesterol levels. Statins act by inhibiting a liver enzyme that generates cholesterol. Bile acid sequestrants, nicotinic acid, and fibrates are among the more cholesterol-lowering drugs.

2. **Blood pressure medications:** Hypertension (high blood pressure) may damage the arteries and raise the chance of having a heart attack or stroke. Angiotensin-converting enzyme (ACE) inhibitors and angiotensin receptor blockers (ARBs) may help reduce blood

pressure. Hypertension is also treated with beta-blockers, calcium channel blockers, and diuretics.

3. **Antiplatelet drugs:** Antiplatelet medications work by making platelets in the blood less sticky, which helps avoid blood clots. The most often used antiplatelet drug is aspirin. Clopidogrel, ticagrelor, and prasugrel are some more antiplatelet medicines.

4. **Anticoagulants:** Anticoagulants, commonly known as blood thinners, aid in the prevention of blood clot formation. Warfarin is the most often used anticoagulant. Dabigatran, rivaroxaban, and apixaban are some more anticoagulants.

5. **Nitrates:** Nitrates aid in the dilation of blood vessels, which helps alleviate chest discomfort (angina). Nitrates are classified as either short-acting (nitroglycerin and isosorbide mononitrate) or long-acting (isosorbide dinitrate).

6. **Medication for heart failure:** Medication for heart failure helps the heart pump more effectively and reduces symptoms of heart failure. Heart failure is routinely treated with ACE inhibitors, ARBs, and beta-blockers. Heart failure is also treated with diuretics, digoxin, and aldosterone antagonists.

7. **Antiarrhythmic drugs:** Antiarrhythmic medications are used to

treat irregular heartbeats
(arrhythmias).
Antiarrhythmic drugs that
are often used include
amiodarone,
procainamide, and
sotalol.
These are only a few of
the drugs available to
treat heart disease. Your
doctor may suggest extra
drugs based on your
specific condition. It is
important to take any
drugs exactly as directed
and to address any
concerns or side effects
with your doctor. You
may help minimize your
risk of a heart attack or
stroke by taking the
proper drugs and making
lifestyle adjustments.

C. Surgical Procedures

Cardiac surgery, also known as cardiovascular surgery, is a medical technique used to treat heart conditions such as coronary artery disease, heart valve disease, and congenital heart abnormalities. It usually consists of a mix of open-heart surgery, which includes opening the chest to provide access to the heart and minimally invasive or catheter-based techniques. Heart surgery is a big treatment with high dangers, but it may also save lives and improve quality of life. The patient's risk factors and current medical state

are assessed at the initial
stage of cardiac surgery.
This comprises
electrocardiograms
(ECGs),
echocardiograms, chest
X-rays, and CT scans.
The patient's lifestyle and
family history are also
considered. To lessen the
chance of additional heart
issues, the doctor may
also prescribe lifestyle
modifications such as
stopping smoking.
The treatment may be
planned after the patient
is judged to be a suitable
candidate for surgery.
The procedure is carried
out under general
anesthesia, which renders
the patient asleep and
unable to feel discomfort.
The surgeon creates an
incision in the chest and

exposes the ribs to get access to the heart during the procedure. The particular technique is determined by the patient's kind of heart condition.

In the case of coronary artery disease, the surgeon may perform a coronary artery bypass graft (CABG), which includes rerouting blood around an arterial blockage. The surgeon may repair or replace the damaged valve in the case of valve disease. The surgeon may repair holes in the heart or replace valves, arteries, or veins to treat congenital heart abnormalities.

After the surgery, the patient is sent to the critical care unit to

recuperate. The healing
period varies according to
the surgery, however, it
usually takes several
weeks. The patient may
need to relax and reduce
their activity during this
period. The doctor will
monitor the patient's
development and offer
instructions for follow-up
treatment.

Cardiac surgery may save
a patient's life if they
have heart problems. It
does, however, carry
hazards such as infection,
blood clots, and stroke.
Before having heart
surgery, it is important to
explore the risks and
advantages with a doctor.
Lifestyle measures, such
as cardiac rehabilitation,
are also used to treat heart
disease. This includes

supervised exercise programs and lifestyle counseling, both of which may aid in improving cardiovascular health and lowering the risk of future heart issues. While there is no cure for heart disease, these therapies may help to slow the course of the condition and improve the quality of life for individuals who suffer from it. It is important to review all treatment choices with your doctor to ensure that you are getting the best care possible for your specific circumstance.

There are various actions you may take, in addition to medical therapy, to minimize your chance of getting heart disease.

They include consuming a balanced diet and exercising regularly, as well as keeping a healthy weight. It is also critical to prevent smoking and excessive drinking, as well as to manage stress. You may help minimize your chance of acquiring heart disease or delay its course if you already have it by following these precautions.

VI. Heart Disease Prevention

Heart disease is one of the main causes of mortality in many nations, therefore it's important to understand the risk factors and how to avoid them.

Understanding the risk factors for heart disease is the first step in avoiding it. High blood pressure, high cholesterol, smoking, obesity, diabetes, physical inactivity, and family history are all risk factors. It is critical to recognize that some of these risk factors are changeable while others are not. Age, gender, and family history are non-modifiable risk variables. Numerous measures may be performed to lower the risk of heart disease after the risk factors have been recognized. The first step is to adjust your lifestyle to lower your risk of heart disease. This includes eating a low-fat, saturated-fat diet, exercising for at least 30 minutes every day, stopping smoking, and lowering stress. Moreover, any medical disorders that might raise the risk of heart diseases, such as high blood pressure, diabetes, and high cholesterol, must be monitored and treated. Apart from lifestyle modifications, it is important to ensure that any medical issues are well handled. This involves taking drugs as recommended, keeping medical appointments, and getting frequent heart disease testing.

HEART DISEASE PREVENTION IN PRACTICE

A. A Well-balanced Diet

A balanced diet is essential for avoiding heart disease and other chronic diseases. A healthy diet rich in fruits and vegetables, lean meats, whole grains, and low-fat dairy products may help lower the risk of developing heart disease and other chronic illnesses.

A healthy diet must include **fruits and vegetables**. They're high in vitamins, minerals, and fiber, and they may help lower your risk of heart disease. Fruits and vegetables should account for at least half of each meal. Fruits and vegetables are also low in calories and fat, making them an excellent option for weight loss.

Consuming a variety of fruits and vegetables every day will help you obtain all of the vitamins, minerals, and fiber your body requires.

A healthy diet should also include **lean proteins**. Fish, poultry, and lean cuts of meat such as chicken or turkey are examples of lean proteins. These proteins have less saturated fat, which may help lower the risk of heart disease. Consuming lean proteins in moderation will help you acquire all of the critical nutrients your body requires without ingesting too much-saturated fat.

Whole grains are another essential component of a balanced diet that may help lower the risk of heart disease. Whole grains have a lot of fiber, which helps lower cholesterol and improve blood sugar levels. Consuming whole grains in moderation may assist to ensure that your body receives all of the critical nutrients it needs.

Low-fat dairy products are also an essential component of a balanced diet. Low-fat dairy products have less saturated fat, which may help lower the risk of heart disease. Skim or 1% milk, low-fat yogurt, low-fat cottage cheese, and low-fat cheese may all be part of a balanced diet. Consuming low-fat dairy products in moderation may help you acquire all of the key nutrients your body requires without ingesting too much-saturated fat.

In addition to having a balanced and nutritious diet, **it is critical to restrict your intake of saturated fat, trans fat, and cholesterol.** Saturated fats, trans fats, and cholesterol have all been linked to an increased risk of heart disease. Reducing your intake of saturated fat, trans fat, and cholesterol may help lower your risk of heart disease.

A balanced diet is essential for avoiding heart disease and other chronic diseases. A healthy diet rich in fruits and vegetables, lean meats, whole grains, and low-fat dairy products may help lower the risk of developing heart disease and other chronic illnesses. In addition to maintaining a nutritious diet, it is critical to restrict your intake of saturated fat, trans fat, and cholesterol. Implementing these easy dietary modifications will help lower your risk of heart disease and other chronic diseases.

B. Consistent Exercise

Regular exercise is an essential component of a healthy lifestyle and may lower the chance of getting heart disease. Exercise helps to strengthen the heart muscle and improves its capacity to properly pump blood. It also helps to minimize risk factors for heart disease, such as high blood pressure, obesity, and diabetes. Walking, running, riding, swimming, or participating in sports are all examples of physical exercise. The idea is to pick something you like and incorporate it into your daily routine. Even 30 minutes of moderate physical exercise on most days of the week may help minimize your chance of getting heart disease.

Exercise improves cardiovascular health by boosting the quantity of oxygen and nutrients reaching your heart and other organs. Your heart rate rises, which strengthens and improves the efficiency of your heart muscle. Exercise also aids in weight management and cholesterol reduction, both of which are important risk factors for heart disease.

The workout provides psychological advantages as well. It can relieve stress and boost mood. Frequent exercise might also help you manage your current health concerns better. Regular exercise has been demonstrated in studies to assist persons with chronic conditions such as diabetes and heart disease.

It is critical to start gently and gradually while starting an exercise regimen. Before beginning any workout regimen, consult with your doctor. Your doctor can assist you in creating a regimen that is both safe and successful for you.

Pay attention to the intensity of your activities while exercising. If you're breathing deeply and your pulse rate is racing, it means you're working hard. Be sure you take a few minutes to relax in between activities.

Be careful to remain hydrated when

exercising. Hydrate well before, during, and after your exercise. If you are exercising vigorously, you should consume a sports drink to restore lost electrolytes and carbohydrates.

While exercising, it is essential to wear appropriate attire and footwear. Select comfortable attire that enables you to move freely. Choose shoes with enough shock absorption and support.

If you are new to fitness, you may think about hiring a personal trainer or enrolling in an exercise class. Working with an expert trainer or teacher will help you remain motivated while also ensuring proper form and technique.

Regular exercise is an essential component of a healthy lifestyle and may lower the chance of getting heart disease. Consult your doctor before commencing any fitness regimen to ensure that it is safe for you. Learn good form and technique by working with a trainer or coach. Choose comfortable clothes and shoes that enable you to move freely. Be hydrated by drinking lots of fluids before, during, and after the activity. You may build a pleasant and safe fitness regimen that can help you minimize your risk of getting heart disease with a little thought and preparation.

C. Preventing Risk Factors

Heart disease is a serious public health issue in the United States and the leading cause of mortality. The good news is that it is entirely avoidable. Smoking, high blood pressure, high cholesterol, diabetes, obesity, and physical inactivity are all risk factors for heart disease. However, minimizing these risk factors will help you minimize your chance of having heart disease.

The first step in avoiding heart disease risk factors is to quit smoking. Smoking is a significant risk factor for heart disease and may raise your chances of having a heart attack or stroke. Smoking cessation may lower your risk of heart disease and improve your overall health.

The second stage is to keep your blood pressure under control. High blood pressure may cause artery hardening and narrowing, which can lead to heart disease. A nutritious diet, frequent exercise, and restricting alcohol use are just a few of the lifestyle adjustments that may help you maintain good blood pressure.

The final step is to keep your cholesterol levels in check. High LDL (bad) cholesterol levels may raise your risk of heart disease, but high HDL (good) cholesterol levels can help protect your heart. A nutritious diet, frequent exercise, and avoiding saturated and trans fats may all help you maintain a good cholesterol level.

The fourth stage is to get your diabetes under control. Diabetes raises your chances of getting heart disease, so it's critical to keep your blood sugar levels under control. Diabetes may be controlled by eating a good diet, exercising frequently, and taking medicines as directed. Maintaining a healthy weight is the sixth stage. Obesity and being overweight raise your chances of having heart disease. Eating a balanced diet and engaging in physical activity on a regular basis will assist you in keeping a healthy weight. Lastly, the sixth stage is to engage in physical activity. Physical inactivity raises your risk of heart disease and may lead to other health issues. Exercise may help you maintain a healthy weight and keep your heart in good working order. Try to make sure you get at least 30 minutes of physical activity on most days of the week. You may lower your chance of acquiring heart disease and improve your overall health by avoiding these risk factors. It is important to consult with your doctor before making any lifestyle changes. Moreover, your doctor can monitor your health and advise you on ways to lower your risk of heart disease.

Lastly, it is critical to take precautions to lower the risk of future heart disease. This includes a nutritious diet, frequent exercise, stopping smoking, and lowering stress. Also, it is critical to maintaining medical checkups and tests for heart disease, as well as any other medical issues that may raise the risk of heart disease.

It is feasible to lower the risk of heart disease and improve overall health by recognizing the risk factors linked with heart disease and taking the appropriate actions to reduce the risk. Prevention is the key to lowering the risk of heart disease, and it is critical to take precautions today to lower the risk in the future.

VII. Conclusion

Heart disease is a prominent cause of mortality in the United States, with one in every four fatalities caused by some kind of heart disease. A variety of variables, including lifestyle decisions, genetics, and other medical disorders, contribute to heart disease. Although it is not feasible to avoid all occurrences of heart disease, efforts may be done to lower the chance of getting the illness. Maintaining a healthy lifestyle is one of the most essential things you can do for your heart. This includes eating a well-balanced diet, exercising frequently, avoiding smoking and excessive alcohol intake, and limiting stress. A diet heavy in fruits, vegetables, whole grains, and lean proteins and low in saturated fat may help minimize the risk of heart disease. Exercise aids in the strengthening of the heart muscle, the reduction of blood pressure, and the improvement of circulation. Stress reduction and good sleep may also help minimize the risk of heart disease. Apart from making lifestyle changes, people should be aware of any family history of heart disease and speak with their doctor about any risk factors they may have. Some persons are predisposed to heart disease because of their age, gender, race, or family history. Understanding the risk factors may help people take precautions and make lifestyle adjustments to enhance their heart health. Moreover, frequent medical visits may aid in the early detection of any indicators of heart disease. Regular checks and discussions with a doctor about any symptoms may help detect any issues early when they are simpler to treat.

Lastly, it is important to be aware of the symptoms of heart disease and to seek medical assistance if any of them occur. The most common symptoms of heart disease are chest pain or discomfort, shortness of breath, arm or shoulder pain, exhaustion, and dizziness. Heart disease is a dangerous disorder that, if left untreated, may lead to life-threatening consequences. Adopting lifestyle adjustments and being aware of potential risk factors may help

lower the likelihood of
acquiring heart disease.
Also, frequent medical
checks and being aware
of the warning symptoms
of heart disease may help
diagnose the issue early
and seek treatment.

Printed in Great Britain
by Amazon

35474688R00069